Doctor Bob's Two Step Program
to
Weight Loss

Easy. Fast. Effective.

Watch Your Weight Take a Nosedive

Robert Rodgers PhD
Zero Point Healers

Contents

Doctor Bob's Two Step Program to Weight Loss

Doctor Bob's Two Step Program to Weight Loss

Seven important questions follow. Record a mental count of the number of yes answers.

1. Are you overweight?
2. Have you tried one diet plan after another with little or no success?
3. Have you succeeded in shedding pounds during the first month of a diet program or exercise routine, but gave up because it was not happening quickly enough?
4. After abandoning one diet program after another do you wind up gaining even more weight than before you began dieting?
5. Looking back on all of your efforts, have they all been futile?
6. Have you tried every weight loss program touted as the best, but none of them helped you lose weight?
7. Are you on a continual hunt for a new program that offers a diet plan or exercise program that is supposed to make it possible to lose weight effortlessly and permanently?

Did you answer "Yes" to four or more of the seven questions above? If so, this book offers the answer you have been searching for: a simple yet powerful approach that provides the foundation for losing weight successfully and permanently.

I must warn you at the outset that Doctor Bob's Two Step Program is not an approach you would have ever expected to encounter. As counter-intuitive and illogical as it may appear at first, my Two Step Program will work for you if you give it a chance.

The Daunting Challenge of Diet Programs

Millions of people are just as frustrated as you with each and every well intended attempt to lose weight. Rest assured you are not alone. Why is it that you and pretty much everyone else who is trying to lose weight do not succeed despite all of your well-intended (and often expensive) efforts?

Doctor Bob's Two Step Program to Weight Loss

Are the diet programs you have tried scams? To be sure, some diet programs are certainly better than others for your body, but I have never encountered a diet program to be a scam. Any diet program will help you shed pounds if you stick to it. The problem is having the discipline and focus to stay on track.

Are the exercise programs you have tried scams? Again, some exercise programs are certainly better than others for the unique requirements of your body. I have also never encountered an exercise program that is a scam. If you can stick to doing the exercises prescribed in any exercise program you will lose weight – even if only a pound every week. Guaranteed. A pound every week adds up to 60 pounds after only two months!

OK, if the difficulty with losing weight is not due to the diet plans you have tried or the exercise programs you have attempted, why in the world can't you and 99% of all the other overweight people lose all the weight your heart desires?

Doctor Bob's Two Step Program to Weight Loss

Face it. You know that people who are overweight have more health problems. Duh. You know that people who are overweight tend to have diabetes and heart disease.

Everyone who is overweight knows on some level what they need to do to lose weight.

- You know the type of food you should eat to lose weight.
- You know you have to exercise.
- You know you have to move your body every day, not just on weekends.

Nope. There are no secrets that reveal what it really takes to lose weight. The weight loss technology has been well established for decades. The research is extensive. So, why is it so blasted difficult to lose weight?

The secret why diet plans and exercise programs rarely succeed is revealed with acknowledgement of an entirely unconscious "No Current" that works against all of your good intentions to lose weight. Next I will explain the difference between the energy that sustains your "No Current" with the energy that inspires your "Yes Current." Then, I will offer my two step solution that deactivates the harmful influence of your "No Current." Once deactivated, the positive influence of your "Yes Current" is freed to express itself. When your "Yes Current" becomes the top dog rather than the underdog the intention to lose weight is no longer obstructed.

The "Yes Current"

You have always been clear about your intention to lose weight or you would not be reading my book in the first place! You know it is in your best and highest good to lose weight. You know …

- Your blood pressure will normalize.
- Your sugar levels will stabilize.
- Your self-esteem will soar to new heights.

- Your ability to navigate through tight passage ways and narrow doorways will become effortless.
- Your body will fit easily into the small seats found on airplanes.

OK - you know all of this is true. You do not need to wait for new research studies to show proof that each of these statements is true and valid in all respects. It is not rocket science.

Your intention to lose weight as embodied in these expectations is a lucid reflection of your "Yes Current." Your "Yes Current" says "Yes" to losing weight. Your "Yes Current":

- Is willing to take whatever steps are necessary to succeed no matter how severe or challenging.
- is the conscious, logical and rational expression of your heart's fondest desire to lose weight.

Doctor Bob's Two Step Program to Weight Loss

- is the divine expression of your supreme intelligence.
- is your primary motivation to experiment with one diet plan after another and one exercise program after another even after confronting one disappointment after another.

The end result has a ring of familiarity. No diet plans and no exercise programs succeed in helping you lose weight. Some plans offer temporary relief. They help you shed a few pounds in the short run. But in the long run, all the fat tissues seem to slap right back onto your belly, hips, arms and legs.

These failures have nothing to do with your desire to succeed. You do want to lose weight. What then is the show stopper? It is the mysterious and unacknowledged existence of your "No Current."

The "No Current"

Guess what? There is a force working within you that you cannot quite put your finger on. This force is your "No Current." It undermines all of your best intentions to lose weight.

Everyone in a body (which happens to be all of us) has a "No Current" that works against the best of our intentions. Ability to detect the presence of your "No Current" is for all practical purposes impossible.

- It is entirely unconscious.
- It is not rational.
- It is not logical.
- It cannot be explained with words.
- It cannot be visualized with pictures.
- It cannot be videotaped.
- It cannot be tasted.
- It cannot be bottled up and corked.

What then is this mysterious "No Current" which winds up being our worst enemy that we do not feel, see or hear? In a nutshell it is the exact opposite of your "Yes Current."

1. It is the unconscious current that runs deep inside your emotional self that does not want to eat healthy food.
2. It is the unconscious current which resides deep inside your subconscious that does not want to exercise regularly.
3. It is the unconscious part of you that may be getting something out of being overweight.

You may have just had a knee jerk reaction to what you just read. Why in the world would anyone want to be overweight unless they are acting in a movie role that requires them to be fat? That is a curiosity that emerges from the logical, rational part of you. Reasons for your "No Current" are hidden deep in the crevices of your soul body, not in the folds of your mind. The reasons are not easily accessed or understood.

The real reason why your efforts to lose weight falter time and time again is because your "No Current" is a devious energy that obstructs all of your best efforts to lose weight. Any and all efforts to lose weight will be undermined until you acknowledge the destructive influence of your "No Current."

Your "No Current" is a destructive energy. Your "Yes Current" is a constructive energy. "No Currents" are far more powerful than "Yes Currents."

"No Currents" can potentially be quieted and subdued in the short run by "Yes Currents." In the long run, "No Currents" always – I repeat always – negate the good intentions that are embodied in your "Yes Currents."

There is an internal battle of sorts between the "No Current" and "Yes Current" which always results in the same outcome. Your "No Current" has access to a machine gun. Your "Yes Current" has access to a water gun. "No Currents" will always win the battle until its destructive influence is acknowledged.

Some people refer to the battle between our "No Current" and "Yes Current" as a duality. We hold many dualities within our psychic throughout our lifetime. The two currents tug intentions in opposite directions.

- Part of us wants to make a lot of money (the "Yes Current"). Part of us wants to be poor (the "No Current").
- Part of us wants to travel and see the world (the "Yes Current"). Part of us wants to stay at home and watch TV (the "No Current").
- Part of us wants to be lose weight (the "Yes Current"). Part of us wants to be overweight (The "No Current").

First Step

If you are serious about losing weight you have to get serious about empowering your "Yes Current" to prevail over your "No Current." One step has to be taken at the outset even before buying into any diet plan or exercise program. You must acknowledge that you (like everyone else) have a "No Current" program running deep within your psyche that has been undermining all of your good intentions to lose weight.

You might well be thinking – wait a minute here.

> *Isn't it always better to maintain a positive attitude rather than fixate on the negative? Certainly there is little positive to be found in the destructive nature of my "No Current"?*

Norman Vincent Peale taught us years ago that positive attitudes always result in positive outcomes. Of course it makes a huge difference to have a positive attitude. Normal was right. But you do not derail your "No Current" by refusing to acknowledge that it exists.

Acknowledging the existence of your "No Current" disables and unplugs its destructive influence. It is this acknowledgement in and of itself that mobilizes all of the resources that are needed to transform the duality of the "No Current" versus "Yes Current" into a singular unity of purpose to lose weight.

Everyone is a self-appointed expert in denial. Most people who are overweight deny the existence of their "No Current." They prefer to fool their egos into believing that experimenting with one diet or another or one medication or another or one surgery or another is the best way to lose weight. They convince themselves that at least they are doing something about being fat. They believe that others are in denial of the health consequences of weight gain, not them.

There is certainly nothing wrong per se with denial. It is an effective strategy we use to trick ourselves into believing we are making good choices. I am not ashamed to admit that I find denial to be very useful at times. Sometimes reality is simply too harsh to endure.

There is a downside to denial. Denying the "No Current" exists does not make it go away. It does not disappear because we refuse to acknowledge it exists.

If the "No Current" remains unacknowledged it will continue to undermine all of your best efforts to lose weight. The first step of Doctor Bob's Two Step Weight Loss Program is simple and easy to complete:

> **Step One: Acknowledge the existence of your "No Current." It destabilizes and misdirects all good intentions to lose weight.**

The "No Current" that undermines your good intentions to lose weight is just like a computer virus that is running in the background of your computer (or smart phone). You write a happy birthday email to a friend on their birthday. Weeks later you learn that your friend never received your birthday greeting. Why not? A computer virus ate your birthday greeting before you even sent it.

A computer virus is no different from a "No Current" that is running deep inside the crevices of your unconscious. Both are nasty devils that are difficult, if not impossible to detect. Both are entirely out of sight and out of mind. Both undercut the best of your intentions to lose weight.

Once you realize and acknowledge that the reason your birthday greetings are not being received by your friends is that your computer has a nasty virus, you can take the necessary steps to get rid of the virus once and forever more. But – if you do not acknowledge your computer has a virus, it will continue to run undetected. It will continue to obstruct any and all emails you attempt to transmit to your friends.

Why might you not realize your computer is infected? You have the mistaken belief that you simply thought in your mind you had written your friend an email greeting – but you never actually transmitted the email. In other words, you falsely convince yourself that you are the problem. The real source of the problem is not the virus that is working underground and undetected.

See the similarity with your own thought patterns? You probably beat up on yourself because you have not been able to stick to a diet plan. It is your fault you are fat.

I disagree. It is not your fault! A "No Current" has been undermining all of your good intentions to lose weight. It functions just like the sneaky viruses that infect computers. The destructive force of your "No Current" will continue to prevail over your "Yes Current" because you have not been aware that they even existed.

You will have no chance of unplugging and terminating the "No Current" program until you acknowledge its existence. How in the world do you acknowledge something that is undermining all of your good intentions to lose weight when it never rears its ugly head? It exists under the radar of detection.

No words are adequate to describe it. Your logical, analytical mind cannot make any sense out of it. It is alive. It functions to undermine all of your best intentions to lose weight.

Emotional Foundations for "No Currents"

The decisive factor that determines whether you succeed with losing weight has nothing to do with diet plans or exercise programs. As noted, most any of them will help you lose weight if you can stick to them. Most people cannot stick to their diets because their "No Current" undermines all of their best efforts.

Doctor Bob's Two Step Program to Weight Loss

Two primary reasons in particular account for why a "No Current" program may have been installed on the hard drive of your inner psyche: Invasion and Abandonment. Perhaps one will call out to you as the primary culprit.

Invasion

- Were you humiliated or ridiculed as a child?
- Do you have a fear of being controlled by others?
- Do you resent it when other people finish the sentences you start but have not yet had a chance to finish?

There it is.

Packing extra pounds on your body creates a cushion between you and other people. The extra weight provides a protective shield. The padding of armor in the form of fat tissue shields you from being controlled and manipulated by other people. After all, you are the bigger one who has the advantage of throwing your weight around.

Doctor Bob's Two Step Program to Weight Loss

Warriors during the Middles Ages used metallic shields to protect against unwanted attacks. We use the same technology today. The only difference is that the body shield we use is composed of fat tissues, not steel. The "No Current" will sustain a thick shield in the form of excess fat until the wound of invasion is healed

Once the fear of being humiliated and controlled is acknowledged people are free to express themselves without anticipating invasion by others. Excess pounds can finally be shed as the fears of control, invasion and humiliation are acknowledged.

Abandonment

- Were you abandoned at an early age?
- Did you fail to receive the nourishment that is the birthright of all children?
- Did your parents give you up for adoption?
- Did your mother feed you with a bottle rather than her breast?

22

- Were your parents poor and unable to put enough food on the table for the family?

There it is.

Every child has a birthright to nourishment by parents. If children to not receive the support from their parents for whatever reason, the child will take on the wound of abandonment until it is acknowledged and healed.

People who were abandoned as children will feel an empty hole deep inside themselves. How can this hole be filled? How can the haunting feeling of emptiness be squelched?

One way is obvious. Habitual and excessive eating serves this purpose quite well indeed, especially when seduced by foods that are yummy to the tummy. So what if they cause weight gain? Certainly it is more useful to fill the hole with something – anything.

Other Reasons That Will Activate a "No Currents"

There are reasons other than invasion and abandonment that can trigger food cravings. Whatever the reason for you, food can prove successful in filling an emotional hole that was never filled as a child.

The pain of having been abandoned or humiliated can be sedated with food for a few minutes or hours, but the pain caused by the emptiness that is felt deep inside the body will resurface time and time again until the feelings are acknowledged and released.

What happened to you? Something has happened to everyone. Completion of Step One simply asks that you acknowledge the existence of your "No Current" whatever the reason may be. If you have made a valiant effort and not succeeded in losing weight, rest assured that you indeed do have a "No Current" program that is running nonstop in your psyche.

If none of the possibilities I have mentioned resonate with you, entertain other possible reasons why your own "No Current" was installed at the soul level. Once you identify a logical reason, you will be in a stronger position to acknowledge the existence of your own unique "No Current" energy.

If you have tried again and again to lose weight without success rest assured your "No Current" is actively undermining all of your best efforts to diet and exercise. While the reason more than likely resides in experiences from your distant past when you were a child, the reason may originate from experiences in the recent past.

Is a family member or friend smothering you, controlling you or humiliating you? One way to feel better under such circumstances is to eat sweets or carbs. Some people prefer other opiates such as alcohol to numb the pain. Alcohol makes people's faces red. Food packs the pounds on. Neither outcome is good for your health.

The preferred choice is to acknowledge the destructive influence of your "No Current." It does not matter a great deal what the reasons for its existence are. What matters is that you acknowledge it exists.

No, you cannot see it. Yes, it is hidden from sight and mind. And yes, it is the singular reason why you have been unsuccessful with losing weight to date.

Acknowledge existence of your "No Current"

When I say acknowledge that your "No Current" exists, that is all you need to do. Acknowledge it! You certainly do not have to remember the hurtful circumstances that gave birth to your "No Current" whether they involved invasion, control, humiliation or abandonment. Years of talk therapy with a psychologist are not necessary. Reliving the past is certainly not in your best and highest good, especially when memories are painful.

Completion of Step one is simple and straightforward. Do it right now. You have nothing to lose but weight.

Step One Summary

Your approach to weight loss so far has been to focus on your "Yes Current." Perhaps you have even formulated affirmations that are inspired by the innate wisdom of your "Yes Current."

> *At this time and in this place, I light a fire under my intention to lose weight. I am disciplined. I am focused. I am determined.*

Sounds great, eh? I applaud your past efforts. There may be a golden tongue to the verbiage, but this approach works against all of your best intentions to lose weight. These affirmations are not working for you are they? You only wind up feeling guilty over and over again because you cannot satisfy your own expectations.

Doctor Bob's Two Step Program to Weight Loss

Why? Your "Yes Current" keeps getting sabotaged by your sneaky "No Current." I say once again – your "No Current" always prevails in the end. If you do not acknowledge the elephant in your own body (which is the "No Current") you will never succeed with cleaning out the turds that have been stinking up all of your best efforts to lose weight. Focusing your thoughts and plans on the "Yes Current" leads to weight gain.

If you are serious about losing weight, turn your approach upside down. Get in touch with the seedy nature of your "No Current." Once you feel into the slimy character of this energy, it will release.

Step One asks that you face up to your "No Current" cheek to cheek, nose to nose and head to head. This is the affirmation that succeeds:

> *At this time and this place I acknowledge the existence of my "No Current". I understand you are the reason I have been*

unable to lose weight. I now know you exist and I am aware you have been hiding out deep inside the silk lining of my soul. Now that I know you exist it is time for you to scram. Find another fat host to pester. I am no longer available.

Acknowledge your "No Current." Weight will begin to slip off your body like an ice cream cone melting on a hot summer day.

Second Step

Now that you have acknowledged the existence of your "No Current" you will most likely want to distance yourself from it.

- Perhaps step aside from all that it entails.
- Perhaps cast away the seeds of experience that gave birth to it.

Doctor Bob's Two Step Program to Weight Loss

The second step of Doctor Bob's weight loss program asks that you do not even attempt to banish the "No Current" from consciousness. Using your will to quiet it will prove a futile exercise. Attempts to squelch your "No Current" infuse it with even more energy. You will top off the level of fuel in its gas tank.

Your "No Current" is much like a child. Ever try to subdue the energy of a child? Your "No Current" reacts just like a child when confronted with demands it be silenced. Both get more defiant and difficult.

You cannot force your "No Current" into submission. You cannot control it. Try to isolate it and it becomes more problematic. Hoping that your "No Current" will fade away into the sunset has as much promise of success as reversing the effects of global warming.

OK. How do you go about taming that fierce, hungry beast of a "No Current" that continues to rattle inside your thoughts and derail the best of your intentions to lose weight? You are not going to believe the answer I am about to offer. I am quite sure it is not what you would have ever expected.

The only way to neutralize the destructive force of your "No Current" is to "flesh out" its nuances by merging with it. You have to become one with it in order to deactivate it. You have to get in touch with its devious manipulations by merging your own will power with 'No Current" consciousness.

The second step of effortless weight loss is actually as simple as the first. The second step asks you to tap into the power and strength of your "No Current." It is where the juice of your life force resides. It is the nuclear heat pump of your body. Do not waste your energy attempting to tackle, silence or subdue its energy.

Step Two: Invite the consciousness of your "No Current" to engulf you.

Doctor Bob's Two Step Program to Weight Loss

How do you do this? You say no to diets and exercise. You say yes to sugar, sweets and chips and feel into the surge of surge that erupts.

Do a little experiment and you will see what I mean. First say out loud:

> *I need to stick to my diet today.*

How much energy does this statement carry? Now say out loud:

> *I am not dieting today, tomorrow or ever.*
> *Diets are stupid inventions of people who*
> *just want to make money off of me.*

OK. Which of the two statements carries more of an energetic charge? Of course it is the second statement, not the first. The first statement has the energetic charge of a microchip.

It is only through saying No to dieting and exercise programs that your "Yes Current" can move to center stage. Once you tap into the dark energy of your "No Current" its force is reduced to the gentle touch of a bee pollinating a rose. The power of your "No Current" is instantly diffused when you feel its destructive force.

I am well aware Step Two seems to be the opposite of what you "should" be doing. Should you really get back on the band wagon of diets and exercise every day? It hasn't worked in the past and it will unlikely succeed now. Why not give Step Two a trial run? What do you have to lose?

This is precisely how your "No Current" is neutralized. You become its best buddy. There is no other way. Once neutralized, your "Yes Current" becomes the boss rather than the servant. When your "Yes Current" is in charge it is no longer being sabotaged by your "No Current." And when this happens you will finally be in a position to lose weight effortlessly no matter what diet plan or exercise program you decide to use. The miracle of all miracles is that no diet plan or exercise program is even necessary once you have tackled your "No Current."

Thoughts that Support Weight Loss

There is a stark difference between the thoughts that promote weight gain and the thoughts that promote weight loss. .

Weight Gain Thoughts

I really should not eat that chocolate éclair right now. It is not one of the items listed in my fresh veggie diet for today. Eating a chocolate éclair would be the supreme violation of my diet. But, you know what? Today is my mother's birthday. I really should celebrate somehow. What better way to honor my mother than to eat that éclair right now? My mother always bought me the most delicious éclairs when I was a child. So, right on. I will eat that éclair today. I can always return to my diet plan tomorrow.

Doctor Bob's Two Step Program to Weight Loss

This rationale should sound very familiar, eh? I have used this same pattern of thinking as a rationale for eating all sorts of junk foods that packed the pounds on my belly. Let's not deceive ourselves. This thinking does not help us lose weight. It only insures that we will find another excuse tomorrow to eat another sweet desert that will pack on even more the pounds. Of course we will always plan on returning to the diet the following day but rarely honor the commitment to ourselves. The cycle is familiar to everything who wants to lose weight.

1. You eat bad food.
2. You promise yourself you will get back on your diet tomorrow.
3. The next day your ego creates a better excuse why you should waiver from your diet.
4. You eat more bad food.
5. You promise you will return to your diet tomorrow.

Tomorrow never comes.

Weight Loss Thoughts

> *Look at that lovely chocolate éclair. There is no doubt about it. That is what my body needs right now. You betcha. I do not care what it does to my body fat. Hell, I need to eat two éclairs today. Chocolate is good for my hormones. Chocolate lifts my sour moods. An éclair is precisely what I need in the moment. Why, my body knows what food it needs and there it is by God. That yummy chocolate éclair is it. I am gulping it down right now.*

Obviously, it is a bad idea to eat the éclair. It will cause weight gain, not weight loss. But admit it. There is a huge difference between the weak energetic charge of weight gain thought patterns and the strong energetic charge of weight loss thought patterns. The former carries little juice and emits a barely audible voice. We are talking the light of candles and the sound of whispers.

Doctor Bob's Two Step Program to Weight Loss

Weight loss thoughts carry a punch that will knock out a heavy weight fighter in the first round. We are talking the force of nuclear power here. A successful diet plan cannot be sustained with feeble minded thoughts. It requires the type of energy that that inspires victory.

The idea behind the Second Step of Effortless Weight Loss is to tap into the charge behind "No Current."

- You do not deny the power.
- You do not attempt to subdue it.
- You do not attempt to lasso it.
- You do not attempt to bleed it to death.
- You do not try and settle it down through manipulation or deception.

None of these strategies will succeed. The gateway to weight loss is to go with the flow of your "No Current." Tap into the energetic charge that pushes you to eat food that makes you fat.

Do not hold back. Do not hesitate. Do not be

ashamed. Do not qualify your thought patterns because your ego tells you that what you are saying and thinking is obviously illogical.

Of course it is not logical. That is why Step Two proves to be so successful for people. It gives you direct access to the illogical reasoning processes that fuel your "No Current."

What really happens when you access the overpowering energy behind the never ending urge to eat foods that are bad for you? A healing happens. You are able to access the unpleasant feelings that trigger food cravings. Instead of thinking you are craving sweets because they taste good or because you have some short circuit in your brain, you are able to access the real reasons for the cravings.

If the real reason for food cravings is abandonment you experienced as a child, you get direct access to that wound. You understand at the visceral level that certain foods fill the hole that was formed from being abandoned at an early age.

Once the feeling is accessed even for a few seconds (in the case abandonment) it is released. The energetic charge that triggers your craving for sweets is defused.

You gain unobstructed access to the energetic charge that fuels food cravings by becoming one with it. You do not fight it. You absorb its energy. Martial artists do just this. They absorb the blows of an opponent.

Once the emotional reasons that underpin food cravings are accessed, emotional holes are magically filled with love and acceptance. Reasons that trigger food cravings vanish. Food as a filer becomes unnecessary.

You may well still want to eat that chocolate éclair but it is because you desire it, not because you are trying to fill up an emotional hole that was formed in childhood.

Doctor Bob's Two Step Program to Weight Loss

Some people are hesitant to access unpleasant feelings from abandonment or invasion for fear that the pattern of excessive eating will intensity. They worry more fat will pack onto their belly. Excessive food cravings are driven by the existence of an emotional hole. Heal the hole and you tame the frantic urge to eat excessively.

Other people fear that Step Two will activate a barrage of horrible memories and hurtful feelings experienced during childhood. When you access the feelings that lie just underneath the food cravings they are released and healed.

Filling the hole does not take years or months or weeks. It can happen instantly. It takes far more energy to run away from the unpleasant feelings than to pause and acknowledge them. Asserting your "no" to dieting plans and your "yes" to sweets and cars is the one authentic way to banish your "No Current" to the garbage dump. This will put your "Yes Current" in charge. It lights a fire under your pure intention to lose weight.

Step Two Summary

If you are serious about neutralizing your "No Current" you do not want to continue saying "yes" to dieting and exercising. That is what you have been trying to do all along. This approach is guaranteed to induce guilt, frustration and failure. The second step of Doctor Bob's weight loss program involves saying not just "No" but "Hell No" to dieting and exercise.

Does this seem counter-intuitive? It should because it is. You have probably been thinking all along that you have to motivate yourself to stick to diets. When you fall off the wagon you get depressed and beat up on yourself for not being enough.

You already know that you (and everyone else trying to lose weight) cannot muster up the focus, dedication and discipline over the long haul to stick with a diet. Such feeble attempts drain your enthusiasm, weaken your spirit and siphon off your life force. Diets do not work now and have never worked in the past. Right? What does work?

Getting acquainted with your "No" infuses your life force with an abundance of energy. It is an interesting and fun experience. You will be delighted to discover that when you tap the consciousness of your "No" you have all the motivation necessary to lose weight.

In short, If you continue to honor your commitment to a diet you will continue to feel guilty about falling short of your own expectations.

> I should be better. I continue to sin. I continue to fall off the wagon. I can't help myself. I am a bad person.

When you try and honor your intention to stick to a healthy diet your "No Current" will win out every time. Your "No Current" runs the show of your life until you bring it out into the open and expose it. Once exposed, the grip it has on you will release. Once acknowledged, "No Current" program is removed from the hard drive of your consciousness. It becomes a mere spectator in the peanut gallery rather than the master in control of your decisions about food.

Your logical self that wants to say "Yes" to diets has no chance of winning the heavyweight fight for your life. Your "No Current" will always be heavier, smarter, craftier, cleverer and sneakier than your "Yes Current" until it is acknowledged (Step One) and disabled (Step Two).

How to Disable Your "No Current"

There are two ways to get in touch with the feelings that energize your "No Current." The first approach is to say "No" to all those diet plans and exercise programs. The second approach is to say "Yes" to foods that cause weight gain.

Say "No" to Diet Plans

Try out this argument for how to resist any and all diet plans.

Does my overextended belly bother you? You are thinking maybe you are better than me because you are "thin"? Well, think that if you want but you are in for a big surprise.

I am here to tell you that the bulge that you see in my belly is a safe storehouse for toxins that have crept into my body. Because I have safely isolated the toxins in my fatty tissues they do not leak into my vital organs. It is for this reason and this reason alone that you are not going to see any toxins in my heart or my lungs. That is because the gorgeous fat cells in my belly have sequestered them. It is a segregation program that keeps my heart pumping and my lungs expanding.

Now, I do not want to worry you unnecessarily, but have you noticed that a lot of thin people in their thirties have heart attacks? Do you know why? It is because their body did not have any way to isolate the deadly toxins. You see, toxins head straight to the vital organs of thin people because the body has no storehouse for them.

Stay thin if you want - but accept the consequences I say. My toxins have been sent to a safe storehouse where they can do no harm to my vital organs. Now that is pretty cool, eh?

Say "Yes" to Sugar and Carbs

You are most likely asking yourself right now ...

If I get in touch with my food cravings won't I just double my weight in a matter of weeks?

45

If I tell myself how good French fries are for my body, won't I just eat more of them and gain even more weight?

Remember the reason for saying "Yes" to all the foods that are bad for you to eat. Doing so is the only way to tap into the destructive energy of your "No Current." Instead of skating across the surface of this unconscious energy and thereby keeping it trapped deep inside your psyche you make the energy conscious by merging with it. When the connection has been made you disconnect its energetic charge and disable its harmful effects.

When you say "Yes" to bad food, you are not being logical or technically correct in any respect. Rather, you tap into that unconscious part of yourself that is working against all of your best intentions to lose weight. Feelings and experiences that were buried alive at a time long ago and in a place far are accessed to be released.

Some of the feelings may well not be pleasant. Allow them to surface anyway. They have been under water for too long.

The most exciting news of all is that once you feel into the consciousness of your "No Current" its charge is defused. Impulses that motivate excessive eating – whether they are due to abandonment or invasion or ridicule or control – will no longer influence your decisions to eat cake, ice cream and candy. You do. When your "Yes Current" becomes the boss, food choices are motivated by a pure intent for pleasure. There is no need to fill an emotional hole.

Blow the Fuse on Your "No Current"

Next I offer some admittedly outrageous examples of how you can access the dark energy of your "No Current" and, in so doing, release it not only now but forever more. Be warned you do have to be outrageous if you are serious about accessing the consciousness of your "No Current."

It is hanging out in the core of your subconscious. Barricades that surround this consciousness are as thick as the walls that guard the gold in Fort Knox (USA).

Keep in mind that the idea behind each outrageous statement is to see only the positive value to foods that will make you gain weight if you eat them regularly. Once you get into the flow and spirit of the Step Two approach, you will be well prepared to create your own statements about why eating bad food in excess is good for you!

I must confess at the outset that when I get into the flow of making these types of outrageous statements I find it to be terribly fun, exhilarating and outrageously funny.

French Fries

I love ordering extra French fries with my burgers. Fries are super foods. They are made of potatoes which grow in the dirt of mother earth. They contain earth energy. Fries are great for grounding and centering. They always help me keep focused at work. When I eat fries at lunch every day I always get perfect performance evaluations.

Ketchup

It is especially important to pour extra ketchup on my fries. Ketchup you see is a vegetable. Not everyone knows this - but it is true. Just ask one of our greatest Presidents - Ronald Regan. He knew everything that is important to good dieting. After all - how in the world could he have become one of our greatest presidents if he of all people did not know a vegetable when he saw one?

Face it, ketchup is a yummy red in color. Any food that is red has to be charged with a buzz of energy that is over the top.

Burgers

Everyone needs to eat at least one fat hamburger every day. Burger meat is protein. Every buddy knows that. Our body needs protein. Hello? Walter Mondale wanted to know where is the beef? It is in my tummy every day, that's where.

Ice Cream

Ice cream is one of those essential daily foods. Think about it. Cows go to all the trouble to make milk so I can eat it. The least I can do is take advantage of their supreme gift to mankind. So what if I just ate three bowls of chocolate ice cream? It is a sin to let good food spoil that cows went to all the trouble to make.

OK - granted. Most ice cream has a little sugar added. Everyone knows cows did not excrete that sugar. Buy hey - maybe you did not hear - Brain need sugar to function. If I starve my brain of sugar, guess what? I can't think straight. I just finished my three bowls of ice cream and right now, my thinking is lucid and straight as an arrow. That, my friend, is because I am smart enough to eat the ice cream that just happens to include the sugar my body so desperately needs. I do not just give purpose to hard working cows. I my brain with the food it needs.

Candy

Have you ever heard people say that candy has no redeeming features? I am here to tell you that happens to be one of those wicked lies perpetuated by internet gossip. The people who keep talking on the internet about how bad candy is for you hide candy bars in the cellars of their houses. They dig it out every day and eat it when no one is looking. You didn't know that? It is true. Put an electronic tracer on them and you will see I am right.

What is up with people who refuse to eat candy? They deny themselves the pleasures of life. They are the people we see every day who do not smile or laugh. They are the people who drag you down into the bottom of the well when you hang out with them because they are so damn depressing. And me? What about me? You are going to have fun when you hang out with me. Good fun. You know why?

I know how to be happy. I know how to have fun. And you know why? It is simple. I know how to have fun because I eat candy - a lot of it.

Chips

Yep - I really like chips. You know why? The salt. My body desperately needs salt. Now, table salt doesn't cut the mustard. The salt that they put in chips has the perfect balance of sodium that my body needs. I get great energy when I eat chips. You want to go around all day long dragging your ass behind your head because you are so tired? That isn't my problem Buddy. Sure I get tired here and there - but a simple hit of a few chips perks me right up. I have all the steam need to clean house, mow the lawn and do my grocery shopping all in one afternoon. One bag of chips does the trick. Of course, if I eat two bags I get even more energy.

So maybe you think chips are a bad idea? Really? Maybe you think chips are not really food? Really? If chips were not food how come I have enough energy to fire a rocket off to the moon?

Chocolate

I eat a lot of chocolate. Yep. And you know why? Chocolate is an antioxidant. That is right big Mamma. Chocolate eats up those nasty free radicals. When free radical buggers get loose in your body all hell breaks loose. I eat at least two chocolate bars a day to make sure those nasty free radicals do not get out of control.

Better yet, chocolate bars balance out my hormones like you would never believe. If I get just a little down in the dumps, one little chocolate bar - or sometimes two – does the trick. It is magical. My mood lifts and am good to go for at two hours and sometimes four hours. If I eat enough throughout the day, I am good to go until midnight.

Bottom Line of Doctor Bob's Two Step Program

Let's face it. Some diet plans are better than others, but they all are complicated in their own unique ways. With some diets you have to count calories of each meal you eat. Really? I am not going to do that. With other diets you have to balance out the foods that are rich in protein with the foods that are rich in fruit. Which foods are rich in proteins again? The list seems changes every week as new scientific studies reveal new results that discredit everything we thought was true yesterday. Is anything we were taught in the past really true today?

Yes, most diets are complicated, but the greater problem is the challenge of sticking to them. I have personally never met anyone who has successfully stuck to the rules of a diet for longer than a few months. There is always a birthday cake or a chocolate bar that needs to be eaten to celebrate an important event.

What happens when the diet plan is violated? You feel yucky inside. You have failed. You have let yourself down. There must be something terribly wrong with you. After all, who wants to be overweight these days? It is certainly not how movie stars get work!

I believe the solution is much simpler than anyone has ever admitted. The reason for overeating is emotional wounding. If you are serious about losing weight, I am suggesting a simple approach. First, you acknowledge the emotional reason for overeating – the existence of your "No Current." Second, merge with its consciousness. You do this by going with the urge to eat food that is bad for you in excess. You make an excess out of behavior that is already excessive.

Once the consciousness that is pushing you to eat more than you should is revealed in all its glory, its hypnotic influence is defused. The punch of its force on your behavior is softened.

If you insist on dancing around the consciousness of your "No Current" it will continue to pollute your thoughts and drive you to excessive eating. Do not dance around it. Dance with it. Allow it to become your dance partner. Get to know it on an intimate basis.

Different labels can be used to describe the consciousness of your "No Current" like the wound of abandonment or the wound of invasion or the wound of control – but in the end, the body can heal all wounds. It is far less draining on your energy to face up to the wounds and invite them to heal than to denial them.

Why not face the challenge of losing weight by having a little fun? It is no fun beating up on yourself because you forget to measure the calories you ate for breakfast. It is fun to rant about how foods like candy cereals, desserts and whipped cream are good for you to eat in excess.

Have a little fun and laugh a lot when you adopt Doctor Bobs Two Step Program to weight loss? Losing weight should not be painful. If should be fun. It should be energizing. Make it so today. I predict you will be surprised to discover how easy it really is to lose weight.

Two steps and only two steps need to be taken. They are simple to do. They are free to take. Best of all, they cost nothing. Why not give Doctor Bob's Two Step Program a trial run? I say it again. You have nothing to lose but weight.